HIGH-PROTEIN HIGH-FIBER MEAL PREP COOKBOOK

Different and Nutritious recipes to create over 700 meals, living a healthy lifestyle with a 31 days meal plan.

Wilbur Avery

INTRODUCTION

Let me introduce you to Susan, a health-conscious person who is determined to feed her body well-balanced meals. Susan, who has a hectic lifestyle and wants to maximize her well-being, has learned about the amazing advantages of eating a diet strong in protein and fiber. Determined to transform her eating habits for the better, she sets out to design a customized meal prep schedule that meets her dietary requirements.

Susan knows there are many benefits to eating a high-protein, high-fiber diet. It not only supplies the necessary building blocks for muscle growth and repair, but it also helps control weight by decreasing cravings and encouraging feelings of fullness. Adding fiber also promotes intestinal health, facilitates digestion, and helps control blood sugar levels.

Susan embarks on an exploration into the realm of meal prep, armed with her enhanced comprehension of the potential of foods rich in protein and fiber. She gains knowledge of the essential components that ensure her meals are satiating and nutrient-dense by packing a punch in terms of protein and fiber. From healthful grains and fiber vegetables to lean meats and legumes, Susan finds a wide range of options to add to her repertoire of foods to prepare meals.

Susan discovers the value of efficient meal preparation methods on her voyage. She learns time-saving techniques that let her plan ahead for meals and stick to a regular eating schedule, like batch cooking and portion control. Equipped with an abundant pantry and an array of wholesome

INTRODUCTION

Let me introduce you to Susan, a health-conscious person who is determined to feed her body well-balanced meals. Susan, who has a hectic lifestyle and wants to maximize her well-being, has learned about the amazing advantages of eating a diet strong in protein and fiber. Determined to transform her eating habits for the better, she sets out to design a customized meal prep schedule that meets her dietary requirements.

Susan knows there are many benefits to eating a high-protein, high-fiber diet. It not only supplies the necessary building blocks for muscle growth and repair, but it also helps control weight by decreasing cravings and encouraging feelings of fullness. Adding fiber also promotes intestinal health, facilitates digestion, and helps control blood sugar levels.

Susan embarks on an exploration into the realm of meal prep, armed with her enhanced comprehension of the potential of foods rich in protein and fiber. She gains knowledge of the essential components that ensure her meals are satiating and nutrient-dense by packing a punch in terms of protein and fiber. From healthful grains and fiber vegetables to lean meats and legumes, Susan finds a wide range of options to add to her repertoire of foods to prepare meals.

Susan discovers the value of efficient meal preparation methods on her voyage. She learns time-saving techniques that let her plan ahead for meals and stick to a regular eating schedule, like batch cooking and portion control. Equipped with an abundant pantry and an array of wholesome

4. Blood Sugar Regulation: Blood sugar levels are positively impacted by both fiber and protein. Protein aids in reducing the rate at which glucose is absorbed, averting abrupt increases in blood sugar. Stable blood sugar levels and better glycemic control can be achieved with the use of fiber, especially soluble fiber.

5. Heart Health: By lowering cholesterol and lowering the risk of cardiovascular illnesses, a high-protein, high-fiber diet can help to maintain heart health. In the digestive system, soluble fiber binds to cholesterol to stop it from being absorbed into the bloodstream.

6. Enhanced Energy: One essential nutrient for the synthesis of energy is protein. It contributes to the creation of hormones and enzymes necessary for metabolism as well as the delivery of oxygen to cells. You may maintain steady energy levels all day long by eating enough protein.

7. Weight management: A diet high in protein and high in fiber can be very helpful in managing weight because of its combination of nutrients. These nutrients help sustain a healthy body weight, decrease hunger pangs, and increase feelings of fullness.

8. Nutrient Density: A diet high in fiber and protein frequently consists of a wide range of foods that are high in nutrients. Your body will acquire the vital vitamins, minerals, and antioxidants it needs to function at its best if you prioritize whole grains, lean meats, fruits, veggies, and legumes.

9. Better Gut Health: Fiber feeds the good gut bacteria by acting as a prebiotic. A high-fiber diet can help with better digestion, nutrient absorption, and general gut health by promoting a healthy gut flora.

10. Long-Term Health Benefits: According to research, eating a diet high in protein and fiber may lessen the risk of developing chronic illnesses like type 2 diabetes, several types of cancer, and cardiovascular disorders.

11. Bone Health: To keep bones strong and avoid diseases like osteoporosis, protein is necessary. It supports strong and robust bones by aiding in the development and repair of bone tissues as well as the absorption of calcium.

12. Boost Metabolism: Protein requires more energy to digest and process than fats or carbohydrates due to its increased thermic impact. Your metabolic rate may rise a little as a result, helping you burn calories and maintain your weight.

Thirteen. Muscle Recovery: Eating a high-protein meal after strenuous exercise or physical activity can aid in the rebuilding and repair of muscle tissue. It offers the essential amino acids required to promote muscle healing and lessen discomfort in the muscles.

14. Hormone Production and Regulation: Proteins are essential for the synthesis and regulation of hormones. Numerous physiological processes, such as mood, hunger regulation, and metabolism, are regulated by hormones. A diet rich in protein helps these hormones work properly.

15. Healthy Aging: As we get older, our muscle mass gradually decreases and our chance of developing chronic illnesses rises. Through the preservation of muscle mass, promotion of healthy aging, and reduction of the risk of age-related muscle loss (sarcopenia), a high-protein, high-fiber diet can help attenuate these consequences.

16. Better Brain Function: Neurotransmitters, which are essential for the best possible brain function, are produced with the help of protein. You can promote mental clarity, focus, and memory by eating enough protein.

17. Reduced Risk of Overeating: It's well known that fiber and protein both boost fullness and curb hunger. Your chances of overindulging in unhealthy snacks or overeating are reduced when you include these nutrients in your meals.

18. Balanced Blood Pressure: Lean proteins and plant-based fibers, in particular, can help to maintain healthy blood pressure levels. A diet high in protein and fiber can also help to achieve this. By doing this, the chance of hypertension and its related cardiovascular problems can be decreased.

19. Enhanced Immune Function: The growth and control of the immune system depend heavily on protein. Consuming enough protein helps the body produce antibodies and immunological cells, which fortify the body's defenses against diseases and infections.

20. General Well-Being: Eating a diet rich in protein and fiber helps promote general well-being. Essential nutrients, stable blood sugar, better digestion, and long-lasting energy can all help one feel more vibrant and optimistic about life.

Including high-fiber items in meal planning is essential to producing wholesome, well-balanced meals. A vital nutrient, fiber supports general health, aids with digestion, and encourages satiety. You may satisfy your daily fiber requirements and take advantage of the many advantages that come with incorporating a range of high-fiber products into your meal planning. When creating your food plan, take into account these top high-fiber ingredients:

1. Whole Grains: Choose whole grains such as whole wheat pasta, quinoa, brown rice, and oats. Unlike processed grains, these grains maintain their fiber-rich bran and germ.

2. Legumes: A great source of dietary fiber are beans, lentils, chickpeas, and other legumes. They can be used as the foundation for flavorful plant-based recipes or as an addition to soups, stews, and salads.

3. Fruits: A lot of fruits are high in dietary fiber. Strawberries, blackberries, and raspberries are berries that are very high in fiber. Oranges, pears, and apples are also great options.

4. veggies: Include a range of veggies in your food plan, including carrots, broccoli, Brussels sprouts, avocados, and leafy greens like kale and spinach. Both soluble and insoluble fiber can be found in these veggies.

5. Chia Seeds: Packed with fiber, these little seeds are a powerhouse. They can be a topping for salads and porridge, or they can be added to yogurt and smoothies.

6. Flaxseeds: You may simply include flax seeds into your meal planning as they are another excellent source of fiber. Ground flaxseeds can be used to baked dishes, salads, and cereals.

7. Nuts and Seeds: A few nuts and seeds that are high in dietary fiber are almonds, pistachios, and sunflower seeds. They can be added to meals for extra flavor and crunch, or they can be enjoyed as a quick and wholesome snack.

8. Bran Cereal: Bran cereals, including oat or wheat bran, have a very high fiber content. Savor it as a cereal for morning or as a garnish for smoothie bowls or yogurt.

9. Whole Grain Bread: To enhance your intake of fiber, choose whole grain bread rather than refined white bread. If you want to add even more fiber, look for alternatives that contain grains or seeds.

10. Psyllium Husk: Psyllium husk is a soluble fiber supplement that can be used to boost the fiber content of baked goods or smoothies.

11. Quinoa: This ancient grain has a high fiber content in addition to being a fantastic source of protein. Quinoa can be added to salads, eaten as a side dish, or even used in place of rice in a number of different dishes.

12. Artichokes: Packed with fiber, artichokes are a tasty vegetable. You can eat them grilled, steamed, or mixed into salads and pasta recipes.

Thirteen. Berries: Berries, including raspberries, blackberries, and blueberries, are rich in fiber and antioxidants. They can be eaten as a healthy snack on their own or as a wholesome addition to yogurt and smoothies.

14. Sweet potatoes: Sweet potatoes include a good quantity of dietary fiber in addition to being a fantastic source of vitamins and minerals. They make a healthy, high-fiber side dish when baked, roasted, or mashed.

15. Brussels sprouts: Packed with fiber and flavor, these little cabbages are also rather healthy. To add extra nutrition to stir-fries and salads, roast them with olive oil and herbs.

16. oats: Eating a bowl of oats first thing in the morning is a great way to get more fiber in your diet. Choose rolled or steel-cut oats, then add berries, almonds, and seeds to boost flavor.

17. Edamame: Young soybeans, or edamame, are a wonderful source of plant-based protein and a good source of fiber. Steamed for a snack, or add them to salads and stir-fries.

18. Popcorn: When cooked with little to no oil or air-popped, popcorn can be a filling and healthful snack choice. This whole grain provides fiber and can be flavored with additional herbs and spices.

19. Cabbage: A vegetable that is high in fiber and adaptable to a variety of cooking methods is cabbage. For further advantages to gut health, try it raw in salads, sautéed as a side dish, or fermented into sauerkraut.

20. Bran Flakes: Eating cereal with flakes is a quick and simple approach to increase your intake of fiber. For a high-fiber breakfast, choose choices with little to no added sugar and serve them with milk or yogurt.

Meal planning using these top high-fiber items guarantees that you get the recommended amount of fiber each day while also enhancing the taste and variety of your meals. Try out new recipes and combos to make scrumptious and nourishing meals that enhance your general health and wellbeing. To ensure maximum digestion and comfort, remember to gradually increase your intake of fiber and pay attention to your body's response.

To taste, add salt and pepper.

Guidelines:
1. Mix the lemon juice, olive oil, minced garlic, dried thyme, dried rosemary, salt, and pepper in a small bowl.
2. Pour the marinade over the chicken breasts and place them in a zip-top bag. After sealing the bag, give the chicken a massage with the marinade. Allow it to steep for a minimum of half an hour and a maximum of four hours in the fridge.
3. Set the grill's temperature to medium-high.
4. Take the chicken out of the marinade and throw away any extra marinade.
5. Cook the chicken breasts on the grill for 6 to 8 minutes on each side, or until they are 165°F (75°C) inside. Depending on the thickness of the chicken breasts, cooking times can change.
6. Before serving, take the chicken from the grill and let it rest for a few minutes. Accompany with your preferred sides, such as a crisp salad or roasted veggies.

Recipe 2:

Balsamic Grilled Chicken Breasts

Information about Nutrition:
- 280 calories each serving
32g of protein
- 6g of carbohydrates
- 14g of fat
- 20 minutes for cooking
- 4 servings per serving

Components:
- Four 6-ounce chicken breasts apiece
- Half a cup of balsamic vinegar
- Two tsp olive oil
- Two minced garlic cloves
- One tablespoon of mustard dijon
- One teaspoon of oregano, dried
To taste, add salt and pepper.

Guidelines:
1. Combine the olive oil, balsamic vinegar, dried oregano, minced garlic, Dijon mustard, and salt & pepper in a small bowl.
2. Pour the marinade over the chicken breasts and place them in a zip-top bag. After sealing the bag, give the chicken a massage with the marinade. Allow it to steep for a minimum of half an hour and a maximum of four hours in the fridge.
3. Set the grill's temperature to medium-high.
4. Take the chicken out of the marinade and throw away any extra marinade.
5. Cook the chicken breasts on the grill for 6 to 8 minutes on each side, or until they are 165°F (75°C) inside. Depending on the thickness of the chicken breasts, modify the cooking time.
6. Before serving, take the chicken from the grill and let it rest for a few minutes. Accompany with quinoa or roasted vegetable side dishes.

Recipe 3:

Grilled Teriyaki Chicken Breasts

Information about Nutrition:

3. Evenly distribute and lightly press the Cajun seasoning mixture onto the chicken breasts.

4. Set the grill's temperature to medium-high.

5. Cook the chicken breasts on the grill for 6 to 8 minutes on each side, or until they are 165°F (75°C) inside. Depending on the thickness of the chicken breasts, modify the cooking time.

6. Before serving, take the chicken from the grill and let it rest for a few minutes. Accompany with grilled vegetables or a serving of coleslaw.

Rice and stir-fried beef

Recipe 1:

Traditional Rice and Beef Stir-Fry

Information about Nutrition:
- 400 calories per serving.
- 28g protein
- 45g of carbohydrates
- 12g of fat
- 25 minutes for cooking
- 4 servings per serving

Components:
One pound (450 grams) of thinly sliced beef flank steak or sirloin
- Two tsp soy sauce
- One spoonful of sauce made from oysters
– One tablespoon cornflour
- Two tablespoons, split between two
- One thinly sliced onion

- Two finely sliced bell peppers (of any color)
- Two minced garlic cloves
- One tsp finely chopped ginger
- Two cups of cooked rice
To taste, add salt and pepper.
- Sliced green onions are an optional garnish.

Guidelines:
1. Mix the cornstarch, oyster sauce, and soy sauce in a bowl. Toss to coat after adding the sliced steak. Give it ten minutes to marinate.
2. In a big skillet or wok, heat up one tablespoon of vegetable oil on high heat.
3. When the skillet is heated, add the marinated meat and stir-fry it for two to three minutes, or until browned. After taking the steak out of the griddle, set it aside.
4. Add the last tablespoon of vegetable oil to the same skillet. Add the grated ginger, minced garlic, bell peppers, and chopped onion. Stir-fry the vegetables for 3–4 minutes, or until they are crisp-tender.
5. To blend all the flavors, throw the cooked meat back to the skillet and stir-fry it for a further one to two minutes. To taste, add salt and pepper for seasoning.
6. Over cooked rice, serve the stir-fried beef. If desired, garnish with chopped green onions.

Recipe 2:

Rice and Teriyaki Beef Stir-Fry

Information about Nutrition:
Calories per serving: 380

- Fresh cilantro, chopped, is an optional garnish.

Guidelines:
1. Mix the cornstarch, rice vinegar, and soy sauce together in a bowl. Toss to coat after adding the sliced steak. Give it ten minutes to marinate.
2. In a big skillet or wok, heat up one tablespoon of vegetable oil on high heat.
3. When the skillet is heated, add the marinated meat and stir-fry it for two to three minutes, or until browned. After taking the steak out of the skillet, set it aside4. Add the last tablespoon of vegetable oil to the same skillet. Add the chopped garlic, grated ginger, broccoli florets, bell pepper, and onion slices. Stir-fry the vegetables for 3–4 minutes, or until they are crisp-tender.
5. To blend all the flavors, throw the cooked meat back to the skillet and stir-fry it for a further one to two minutes. To taste, add salt and pepper for seasoning.
6. Over cooked rice, serve the stir-fried beef with ginger. If desired, garnish with freshly cut cilantro.

Recipe 4:

Rice and Mongolian Beef Stir-Fry

Information about Nutrition:
Calories per serving: 420
26g of protein
- 52g of carbohydrates
- 12g of fat
- 30 minutes for cooking
- 4 servings per serving

Components:
One pound (450 grams) of thinly sliced beef flank steak or sirloin
- One-half cup soy sauce
- Two tsp hoisin sauce
– Two tsp of brown sugar
– One tablespoon cornflour
- Two tablespoons, split between two
- One thinly sliced onion
- Two sliced green onions
- Two minced garlic cloves
- One tsp finely chopped ginger
- Two cups of cooked rice
Garnish options include chopped green onions and sesame seeds.

Guidelines:

1. Mix the soy sauce, hoisin sauce, brown sugar, and cornstarch together in a bowl. Toss to coat after adding the sliced steak. Give it fifteen minutes to marinate.

2. In a big skillet or wok, heat up one tablespoon of vegetable oil on high heat.

3. When the skillet is heated, add the marinated meat and stir-fry it for two to three minutes, or until browned. After taking the steak out of the griddle, set it aside.

4. Add the last tablespoon of vegetable oil to the same skillet. Add the grated ginger, minced garlic, sliced onions, and green onions. Add the onions and stir-fry for 2 to 3 minutes, or until transparent.

5. Add any leftover marinade to the skillet with the cooked steak. To fully incorporate all of the flavors, stir-fry for an extra one to two minutes.

6. Over cooked rice, serve the stir-fried Mongolian meat. If desired, garnish with chopped green onions and sesame seeds.

Curry with lentils and vegetables

Recipe 1:

Vegetable and Lentil Curry

Information about Nutrition:
- 300 calories each serving
12g of protein
- 40g of carbohydrates
- 10g of fat
- 40 minutes for cooking
- 4 servings per serving

Components:
- One cup of rinsed and drained dried lentils (red or green).
- One tablespoon of olive oil
- One chopped onion
- Two minced garlic cloves
1-Tbsp finely chopped ginger
- One teaspoon of cumin powder
- One teaspoon of coriander powder
- One teaspoon of turmeric
One tsp of paprika
- One teaspoon of curry powder
- One 14-oz can of diced tomatoes
- One 14-ounce can of coconut milk
- Two cups of finely cut veggies, such as zucchini, bell peppers, and carrots

To taste, add salt and pepper.
- To garnish, fresh cilantro
- Naan bread or cooked rice ready to eat

Guidelines:
1. Boil four cups of water in a large pot. Cook the lentils for 15 to 20 minutes, or until they become soft. After draining, set away.
2. Heat the vegetable oil in the same pot over medium heat. When the onion is transparent, add the chopped onion and sauté it.
3. Toss in the grated ginger, cumin, coriander, turmeric, paprika, minced garlic, and curry powder. To unleash the flavors, stir thoroughly and simmer for an additional two minutes.
4. Add the coconut milk and diced tomatoes with their juices. Mix everything together.
5. To the pot, add the cooked lentils and chopped vegetables. To taste, add salt and pepper for seasoning.
6. After lowering the heat to a simmer and covering the pot, cook the vegetables for 15 to 20 minutes, or until they are soft and the flavors have combined.
7. Serve the vegetable and lentil curry with naan bread or over cooked rice. Add fresh cilantro as a garnish.

Recipe 2:

Hot Curry with Lentils and Vegetables

Information about Nutrition:
320 calories each serving
14g of protein
- 42g of carbohydrates

- 12g of fat
- 45 minutes for cooking
- 4 servings per serving

Components:
- One cup of washed and drained dried lentils (red or green).
- Two tablespoons olive oil
- One chopped onion
- Two minced garlic cloves
1-Tbsp finely chopped ginger
- One spoonful of curry powder
- One teaspoon of cumin powder
- One teaspoon of coriander powder
- Half a teaspoon, or according to taste, cayenne pepper
- One 14-oz can of chopped tomatoes
- One 14-ounce can of coconut milk
- Two cups of finely cut veggies, such as peas, carrots, and cauliflower
To taste, add salt and pepper.
- To garnish, fresh cilantro
- Naan bread or cooked rice ready to eat

Guidelines:
1. Boil four cups of water in a large pot. Cook the lentils for 15 to 20 minutes, or until they become soft. After draining, set away.
2. Heat the vegetable oil in the same pot over medium heat. Whcn thc onion is transparent, add the chopped onion and sauté it.
3. To the pot, add the grated ginger, minced garlic, curry powder, cumin, coriander, and cayenne pepper. To unleash the flavors, stir thoroughly and simmer for an additional two minutes.
4. Add the coconut milk and diced tomatoes with their juices. Mix everything together.

5. To the pot, add the cooked lentils and chopped vegetables. To taste, add salt and pepper for seasoning.

6. After the vegetables are soft and the curry has thickened, lower the heat to low, cover the pot, and simmer for 20 to 25 minutes.

7. Serve the hot curry of lentils and vegetables with naan bread or over cooked rice. Add fresh cilantro as a garnish.

Recipe 3:

Curry with Coconut Lentil and Vegetables

Information about Nutrition:
- 350 calories each serving
- 10g of protein
- 45g of carbohydrates
- 15g of fat
- 50 minutes for cooking
- 4 servings per serving

Components:
- One cup of washed and drained dried lentils (red or green).
- Two tablespoons olive oil
- One chopped onion
- Two minced garlic cloves
1-Tbsp finely chopped ginger
- One spoonful of curry powder
- One teaspoon of cumin powder
- One teaspoon of ground turmeric
- One 14-oz can of chopped tomatoes
- One 14-ounce can of coconut milk

- Two cups of finely chopped veggies, such as bell peppers, sweet potatoes, and spinach
To taste, add salt and pepper.
- To garnish, fresh cilantro
- Naan bread or cooked rice ready to eat

Guidelines:
1. Boil four cups of water in a large pot. Cook the lentils for 15 to 20 minutes, or until they become soft. After draining, set away.
2. Heat the vegetable oil in the same pot over medium heat. When the onion is transparent, add the chopped onion and sauté it.
3. To the pot, add the turmeric, cumin, curry powder, and grated ginger, minced garlic. To unleash the flavors, stir thoroughly and simmer for an additional two minutes.
4. Add the coconut milk and diced tomatoes with their juices. Mix everything together.
5. To the pot, add the cooked lentils and chopped vegetables. To taste, add salt and pepper for seasoning.
6. After the vegetables are soft and the curry has thickened, lower the heat to low, cover the pot, and simmer for 25 to 30 minutes.
7. Serve the vegetable and coconut lentil curry with naan bread or over cooked rice. Add fresh cilantro as a garnish.

Recipe 4:

Spinach-Vegetable Lentil Curry

Information about Nutrition:
- 280 calories each serving
- 11g of protein

- 38g of carbohydrates
- 9g of fat
- 35 minutes for cooking
- 4 servings per serving

Components:
- One cup of washed and drained dried lentils (red or green).
- One tablespoon of olive oil
- One chopped onion
- Two minced garlic cloves
1-Tbsp finely chopped ginger
- One teaspoon of cumin powder
- One teaspoon of coriander powder
- Half a teaspoon of turmeric
One-half tsp paprika
- One 14-oz can of chopped tomatoes
- Two cups of finely cut veggies, such as potatoes, broccoli, and carrots
- Two cups of raw spinach
To taste, add salt and pepper.
- To garnish, fresh cilantro
- Naan bread or cooked rice ready to eat

Guidelines:
1. Boil four cups of water in a large pot. Cook the lentils for 15 to 20 minutes, or until they become soft. After draining, set away.
2. Heat the vegetable oil in the same pot over medium heat. When the onion is transparent, add the chopped onion and sauté it.
3. To the pot, add the grated ginger, cumin, coriander, turmeric, and paprika along with the minced garlic. To unleash the flavors, stir thoroughly and simmer for an additional two minutes.
4. Add the diced tomatoes together with their liquids and simmer.

5. To the pot, add the cooked lentils and chopped vegetables. To taste, add salt and pepper for seasoning.

6. Simmer until the vegetables are soft, 10 to 15 minutes.

7. Add the fresh spinach leaves and simmer, stirring, until the spinach wilts, about 2 minutes more.

8. Serve the vegetable and lentil curry with naan bread or over cooked rice. Add fresh cilantro as a garnish.

Paella with chicken and shrimp

Recipe 1:

Traditional Paella with Chicken and Shrimp

Information about Nutrition:
- 400 calories per serving.
25g of protein
- 40g of carbohydrates
- 15g of fat
– Prep Time: 60 minutes
- 4 servings per serving

Components:
- Two tsp olive oil
- One chopped onion
- Three minced garlic cloves
- One sliced red bell pepper
- One diced green bell pepper
- Two skinless, boneless chicken breasts, sliced into small pieces
Half a pound of peeled and deveined shrimp

– One cup rice, Arborio
One tsp of paprika
– 1/2 teaspoon of threads of saffron
- Half a teaspoon of oregano, dry
- One 14-oz can of chopped tomatoes
- Three cups of chicken stock
To taste, add salt and pepper.
- To garnish, fresh parsley
- Serving wedges of lemon

Guidelines:
1. Heat the olive oil in a sizable skillet or paella pan over medium heat. Add the chopped bell peppers, minced garlic, and diced onion. Sauté the veggies till they get tender.
2. Place the chicken pieces in the pan and push the vegetables to one side. Cook until each side has a golden brown color.
3. Add the shrimp after moving the chicken to one side of the pan. Cook until they are cooked through and turn pink. After taking the shrimp out of the pan, set it aside.
4. Add the dried oregano, paprika, saffron threads, and Arborio rice to the same pan. Coat the rice in the spices by giving it a good stir.
5. Add the chicken stock and diced tomatoes with their juices. Mix everything together.
6. After bringing the mixture to a boil, turn down the heat. Once the rice is done and has absorbed the liquid, cover the pan and simmer for 30 to 40 minutes.
7. To taste, add salt and pepper for seasoning. Add the cooked shrimp and stir.
8. After taking the pan off the burner, give it five minutes to rest.
9. Serve the shrimp and chicken paella with lemon wedges as a garnish and sprinkle with fresh parsley.

Recipe 2:

Hot Shrimp and Chicken Paella

Information about Nutrition:
Calories per serving: 420
26g of protein
- 42g of carbohydrates
- 16g of fat
– Prep Time: 60 minutes
- 4 servings per serving

Components:
- Two tsp olive oil
- One chopped onion
- Three minced garlic cloves
- One sliced red bell pepper
- One diced green bell pepper
- Two skinless, boneless chicken thighs, diced into small pieces
Half a pound of peeled and deveined shrimp
– One cup rice, Arborio
- One tsp of paprika with smoke
- One-half teaspoon of cayenne
One-half tsp dried thyme
- One 14-oz can of chopped tomatoes
- Three cups of chicken stock
To taste, add salt and pepper.
- To garnish, fresh cilantro
- To serve, lime wedges

Guidelines:
1. Heat the olive oil in a sizable skillet or paella pan over medium heat. Add the chopped bell peppers, minced garlic, and diced onion. Sauté the veggies till they get tender.
2. Place the chicken pieces in the pan and push the vegetables to one side. Cook until each side has a golden brown color.
3. Add the shrimp after moving the chicken to one side of the pan. Cook until they are cooked through and turn pink. After taking the shrimp out of the pan, set it aside.
4. In the same pan, add the Arborio rice, smoked paprika, cayenne pepper, and dried thyme. Coat the rice in the spices by giving it a good stir.
5. Add the chicken stock and diced tomatoes with their juices. Mix everything together.
6. After bringing the mixture to a boil, turn down the heat. Once the rice is done and has absorbed the liquid, cover the pan and simmer for 30 to 40 minutes.
7. To taste, add salt and pepper for seasoning. Add the cooked shrimp and stir.
8. After taking the pan off the burner, give it five minutes to rest.
9. Garnish with fresh cilantro and serve the spicy chicken and shrimp paella with lime wedges.

Recipe 3:

Lemon Garlic Chicken and Shrimp Paella

Information about Nutrition:
- Calories: 410 per serving
- Protein: 24g

- Carbohydrates: 41g
- Fat: 17g
– Prep Time: 60 minutes
- 4 servings per serving

Components:
- Two tsp olive oil
- One chopped onion
- Three minced garlic cloves
- 1 red bell pepper,diced
- One diced green bell pepper
- Two skinless, boneless chicken breasts, sliced into small pieces
Half a pound of peeled and deveined shrimp
– One cup rice, Arborio
- Zest of 1 lemon
- 2 teaspoons lemon juice
- A teaspoon of thyme, dried
- 1/2 teaspoon smoked paprika
- One 14-oz can of chopped tomatoes
- Three cups of chicken stock
To taste, add salt and pepper.
- To garnish, fresh parsley
- Serving wedges of lemon

Guidelines:
1. Heat the olive oil in a sizable skillet or paella pan over medium heat. Add the diced onion and minced garlic. Sauté the veggies till they get tender.
2. Add the diced bell peppers and continue to sauté for another 2-3 minutes.
3. Place the chicken pieces in the pan and push the vegetables to one side. Cook until each side has a golden brown color.

4. Add the shrimp after moving the chicken to one side of the pan. Cook until they are cooked through and turn pink. After taking the shrimp out of the pan, set it aside.

5. In the same pan, add the Arborio rice, lemon zest, lemon juice, dried thyme, and smoked paprika. Stir well to coat the rice with the seasonings.

6. Add the chicken stock and diced tomatoes with their juices. Mix everything together.

7. After bringing the mixture to a boil, turn down the heat. Once the rice is done and has absorbed the liquid, cover the pan and simmer for 30 to 40 minutes.

8. To taste, add salt and pepper for seasoning. Add the cooked shrimp and stir.

9. After taking the pan off the burner, give it five minutes to rest.

10. Serve the lemon garlic chicken and shrimp paella with lemon wedges as garnish. Garnish with fresh parsley.

Recipe 4:

Herb-Roasted Paella with Shrimp and Chicken

Information about Nutrition:
Calories per serving: 420
25g of protein
- 40g of carbohydrates
- 18g of fat
– Prep Time: 60 minutes
- 4 servings per serving

Components:
- Two tsp olive oil

- One chopped onion
- Three minced garlic cloves
- One sliced red bell pepper
- One diced green bell pepper
- Two skinless, boneless chicken thighs, diced into small pieces
Half a pound of peeled and deveined shrimp
– One cup rice, Arborio
- One tsp of dried rosemary
- A teaspoon of thyme, dried
- One-half tsp smoked paprika
- One 14-oz can of chopped tomatoes
- Three cups of chicken stock
To taste, add salt and pepper.
- Fresh basil for decorating

Guidelines:
1. Heat the olive oil in a sizable skillet or paella pan over medium heat. Add the minced garlic and chopped onion. Sauté the veggies till they get tender.
2. After adding the chopped bell peppers, sauté for an additional two to three minutes.
3. Place the chicken pieces in the pan and push the vegetables to one side. Cook until each side has a golden brown color.
4. Add the shrimp after moving the chicken to one side of the pan. Cook until they are cooked through and turn pink. After taking the shrimp out of the pan, set it aside.
5. Add the smoked paprika, dried thyme, dried rosemary, and Arborio rice to the same pan. Toss the rice thoroughly to distribute the spices and herbs.
6. Add the chicken stock and diced tomatoes with their juices. Mix everything together.

7. After bringing the mixture to a boil, turn down the heat. Once the rice is done and has absorbed the liquid, cover the pan and simmer for 30 to 40 minutes.

8. To taste, add salt and pepper for seasoning. Add the cooked shrimp and stir.

9. After taking the pan off the burner, give it five minutes to rest.

10. Serve the paella with prawns and herb-roasted chicken after sprinkling it with fresh basil leaves.

Stew made with beef and vegetables

Recipe 1:

Traditional Beef and Veggie Stew

Information about Nutrition:
- 350 calories each serving
25g of protein
- 30g of carbohydrates
- 12g of fat
Preparation Time: Two hours
- 6" serving size

Components:
- Two pounds of cubed beef stew meat
- Two tsp olive oil
- One chopped onion
- Three minced garlic cloves
- Three carrots, cut and peeled

- Three potatoes, diced and peeled
- Two chopped celery stalks
- One 14-oz can of chopped tomatoes
– Four cups of broth made from meat.
- A teaspoon of thyme, dried
- One tsp of dried rosemary
To taste, add salt and pepper.
- To garnish, fresh parsley

Guidelines:
1. Heat the olive oil in a big pot or Dutch oven over medium heat. Brown the beef stew meat on all sides after adding it. After taking the steak out of the pot, set it aside.
2. Add the minced garlic and chopped onion to the same pot. The onion should be sautéed until transparent.
3. Add the potatoes, celery, and carrots to the pot. After a few minutes, stir and continue cooking until the vegetables begin to soften.
4. Add the diced tomatoes with their juices and the beef stock to the pot with the beef once again. Mix everything together.
5. To the pot, add the dried rosemary and thyme. To taste, add salt and pepper for seasoning.
6. After bringing the stew to a boil, turn down the heat. When the beef is soft and the flavors have combined, cover the saucepan and boil it for one to two hours, stirring now and then.
7. If needed, adjust the seasoning. Serve hot classic beef and vegetable stew with a fresh parsley garnish.

Recipe 2:

Beef and Vegetable Stew Made Slowly

Information about Nutrition:
320 calories each serving
23g of protein
- 28g of carbohydrates
- 10g of fat
- Prep Time: 6 to 8 hours
- 6" serving size

Components:
- Two pounds of cubed beef stew meat
- Two tsp olive oil
- One chopped onion
- Three minced garlic cloves
- Three carrots, cut and peeled
- Three potatoes, diced and peeled
- Two chopped celery stalks
- One 14-oz can of chopped tomatoes
– Four cups of broth made from meat.
- A teaspoon of thyme, dried
- One tsp of dried rosemary
To taste, add salt and pepper.
- To garnish, fresh parsley

Guidelines:
1. In a big skillet set over medium-high heat, warm the olive oil. Brown the beef stew meat on all sides after adding it. The beef should be moved to a slow cooker.
2. Add the minced garlic and chopped onion to the same skillet. The onion should be sautéed until transparent.

3. To the skillet, add the potatoes, celery, and carrots. After a few minutes, stir and continue cooking until the vegetables begin to soften.

4. Add the vegetables and beef to the slow cooker.

5. Add the beef broth and diced tomatoes with their juices. Mix everything together.

6. To the slow cooker, add the dried thyme and dried rosemary. To taste, add salt and pepper for seasoning.

7. Once the meat is soft and the flavors have combined, cover the slow cooker and cook it on low heat for 6 to 8 hours or on high heat for 4 to 6 hours.

8. If needed, adjust the seasoning. Serve the hot beef and vegetable stew from the slow cooker garnished with fresh parsley.

Recipe 3:

Vegetable Stew with Chunky Beef

Information about Nutrition:
Calories per serving: 380
26g of protein
- 32g of carbohydrates
- 14g of fat
Preparation Time: 2.5 hours
- 6" serving size

Components:
- Two pounds of cubed beef stew meat
- Two tsp olive oil
- One chopped onion
- Three minced garlic cloves

- Three carrots, cut and peeled
- Three potatoes, diced and peeled
- Two parsnips, cut and peeled
- Two chopped celery stalks
- One 14-oz can of chopped tomatoes
– Four cups of broth made from meat.
- One spoonful of pasted tomatoes
- A teaspoon of thyme, dried
- One tsp of dried rosemary
To taste, add salt and pepper.
- To garnish, fresh parsley

Guidelines:
1. In a big pot or Dutch oven, warm the olive oil over medium heat. Brown the beef stew meat on all sides after adding it. After taking the steak out of the pot, set it aside.
2. Add the minced garlic and chopped onion to the same pot. Cook the onion until it turns transparent.
3. To the pot, add the celery, parsnips, potatoes, and carrots. After a few minutes, stir and continue cooking until the vegetables begin to soften.
4. Put the diced tomatoes (with their juices), tomato paste, and beef broth back into the pot with the beef. Mix everything together.
5. To the pot, add the dried rosemary and thyme. To taste, add salt and pepper for seasoning.
6. After bringing the stew to a boil, turn down the heat. Once the flavors have combined and the beef is soft, simmer it for two to three hours while covering the pot and stirring now and then.
7. If needed, adjust the seasoning. Garnish the thick beef and vegetable stew with fresh parsley and serve hot.

Recipe 4:

Vegetable and Beef Stew

Information about Nutrition:
- 300 calories each serving
24g of protein
- 26g of carbohydrates
- 9g of fat
Preparation Time: Two hours
- 6" serving size

Components:
- Two pounds of cubed lean beef stew meat
- Two tsp olive oil
- One chopped onion
- Three minced garlic cloves
- Three carrots, cut and peeled
- Three cups of peeled and cubed butternut squash
- Two chopped celery stalks
- One 14-oz can of chopped tomatoes without additional salt
– 4 cups beef broth reduced in sodium
- A teaspoon of thyme, dried
- One tsp of dried rosemary
To taste, add salt and pepper.
- To garnish, fresh parsley

Guidelines:
1. Heat the olive oil in a big pot or Dutch oven over medium heat. Brown the lean beef stew meat on all sides after adding it. After taking the steak out of the pot, set it aside.

2. Add the minced garlic and chopped onion to the same pot. The onion should be sautéed until transparent.

3. Stir in the celery, butternut squash, and carrots. After a few minutes, stir and continue cooking until the vegetables begin to soften.

4. Put the diced tomatoes and their liquids back into the pot together with the low-sodium beef broth after returning the beef to it. Mix everything together.

5. To the pot, add the dried rosemary and thyme. To taste, add salt and pepper for seasoning.

6. After bringing the stew to a boil, turn down the heat. When the beef is soft and the flavors have combined, cover the saucepan and boil it for one to two hours, stirring now and then.

7. If needed, adjust the seasoning. Warm up the nutritious stew of meat and vegetables and sprinkle with fresh parsley.

Marsala chicken

Recipe 1:

Traditional Marsala Chicken

Information about Nutrition:
- 350 calories each serving
- 30g of protein
- 15g of carbohydrates
- 15g of fat
- 30 minutes for cooking
- 4 servings per serving

Components:

- Four skinless and boneless chicken breasts
To taste, add salt and pepper.
- Half a cup of whole wheat flour
- Four tsp unsalted butter
- Two tsp olive oil
- Eight ounces of chopped mushrooms
- Two minced garlic cloves
- One cup of wine, Marsala
- One cup of chicken stock
– 1/4 cup heavy cream
- To garnish, fresh parsley

Guidelines:
1. Add salt and pepper to the chicken breasts for seasoning. Shake off any extra flour after you've coated them.
2. Melt two tablespoons of butter and one tablespoon of olive oil in a big skillet over medium heat. When the chicken breasts are golden brown and well cooked, add them and cook for about 5 minutes on each side. After removing it from the skillet, set the chicken aside.
3. Add the remaining butter and olive oil to the same skillet. When the mushrooms are soft and caramelized, add the garlic and continue to sauté.
4. Add the chicken broth and Marsala wine. After bringing the mixture to a simmer, let it cook for around five minutes to let the alcohol evaporate.
5. After adding the heavy cream, simmer the sauce for a further two to three minutes, or until it slightly thickens.
6. After putting the chicken breasts back in the skillet, cover them with sauce. To fully cook the chicken, cook it for a further two to three minutes.
7. Serve the traditional chicken Marsala hot, topped with a fresh parsley garnish and sauce.

Recipe 2:

Nutritious Marsala Chicken

Information about Nutrition:
- 280 calories each serving
28g of protein
- 10g of carbohydrates
- 12g of fat
- 30 minutes for cooking
- 4 servings per serving

Components:
- Four skinless and boneless chicken breasts
To taste, add salt and pepper.
– 1/4 cup flour (whole wheat)
- Two tsp olive oil
- Eight ounces of chopped mushrooms
- Two minced garlic cloves
- One cup chicken broth with minimal sodium
- One cup of wine, Marsala
– One tablespoon cornflour
- To garnish, fresh parsley

Guidelines:
1. Add salt and pepper to the chicken breasts for seasoning. Shake off any excess whole wheat flour after dredging them in it.
2. Heat the olive oil in a big skillet over medium heat. When the chicken breasts are golden brown and well cooked, add them and cook for about 5 minutes on each side. After removing it from the skillet, set the chicken aside.

3. Add the garlic and mushrooms to the same skillet. Sauté the mushrooms until they become soft.

4. Mix the cornstarch, Marsala wine, and chicken stock in a small bowl until well combined. Transfer the blend into the skillet containing the mushrooms.

5. Simmer the mixture until the sauce thickens, stirring all the while.

6. After putting the chicken breasts back in the skillet, cover them with sauce. To fully cook the chicken, cook it for a further two to three minutes.

7. Spoon the sauce over the chicken and serve the nutritious chicken Marsala hot, garnished with fresh parsley.

Recipe 3:

Creamy Marsala Chicken

Information about Nutrition:
- 400 calories per serving.
32g of protein
- 15g of carbohydrates
- 20g fat
- 40 minutes for cooking
- 4 servings per serving

Components:
- Four skinless and boneless chicken breasts
To taste, add salt and pepper.
- Half a cup of whole wheat flour
- Four tsp unsalted butter
- Two tsp olive oil
- Eight ounces of chopped mushrooms

- Two minced garlic cloves
- One cup of wine, Marsala
- One cup of chicken stock
- One cup thick cream
- To garnish, fresh parsley

Guidelines:

1. Add salt and pepper to the chicken breasts for seasoning. Shake off any extra flour after you've coated them.

2. Melt two tablespoons of butter and one tablespoon of olive oil in a big skillet over medium heat. When the chicken breasts are golden brown and well cooked, add them and cook for about 5 minutes on each side. After removing it from the skillet, set the chicken aside.

3. Add the remaining butter and olive oil to the same skillet. When the mushrooms are soft and caramelized, add the garlic and continue to sauté.

4. Add the chicken broth and Marsala wine. Allow the alcohol to evaporate by simmering and cooking the liquid for approximately five minutes.

5. After adding the heavy cream, simmer the sauce for a further five minutes, or until it thickens.

6. Pour the creamy sauce over the chicken breasts once more and place them back in the skillet. To fully cook the chicken, cook it for a further two to three minutes.

7. Serve the hot, creamy chicken Marsala with a fresh parsley garnish and the sauce spooned over the chicken.

Recipe 4:

Simple and Quick Marsala Chicken

Information about Nutrition:

320 calories each serving

26g of protein

- 12g of carbohydrates

- 16g of fat

- 20 minutes for cooking

- 4 servings per serving

Components:

- Four skinless and boneless chicken breasts

To taste, add salt and pepper.

– 1/4 cup flour (all-purpose)

- Two tsp olive oil

- Eight ounces of chopped mushrooms

- Two minced garlic cloves

- One cup of wine, Marsala

- One cup of chicken stock

- Two teaspoons of butter

- To garnish, fresh parsley

Guidelines:

1. Add salt and pepper to the chicken breasts for seasoning. Shake off any extra flour after you've coated them.

2. Heat the olive oil in a big skillet over medium heat. When the chicken breasts are golden brown and well cooked, add them and cook for about 5 minutes on each side. After removing it from thc skillet, set the chicken aside.

3. Add the garlic and mushrooms to the same skillet. Sauté the mushrooms until they become soft.

4. Add the chicken broth and Marsala wine. After bringing the mixture to a simmer, let it cook for around five minutes to let the alcohol evaporate.

5. Add the butter and stir until it melts and blends thoroughly with the sauce.

6. After putting the chicken breasts back in the skillet, cover them with sauce. To fully cook the chicken, cook it for a further two to three minutes.

7. Serve the quick and simple chicken Marsala hot, topped with a fresh parsley garnish and sauce.

Barley and lentil soup

Recipe 1:

Traditional Barley and Lentil Soup

Information about Nutrition:
- 250 calories per serving.
12g of protein
- 45g of carbohydrates
- Fat: 2 g
- One and a half hours for cooking
- 6" serving size

Components:
- One cup of rinsed green lentils
- 1/2 cup of barley pearls
- One chopped onion
- 2 sliced carrots
- Two sliced celery stalks
- Three minced garlic cloves

– Six cups broth made of vegetables
- A teaspoon of thyme, dried
- One teaspoon of oregano, dried
To taste, add salt and pepper.
- To garnish, fresh parsley

Guidelines:
1. Lentils, barley, celery, carrots, onion, garlic, vegetable broth, thyme, and oregano should all be combined in a big saucepan. Over high heat, bring the mixture to a boil.
2. Once the lentils and barley are soft, reduce the heat to low, cover the pot, and simmer for one hour.
3. Add salt and pepper to taste when preparing the soup.
4. Spoon soup into bowls; sprinkle with parsley, if desired.
5. Warm up this traditional lentil and barley soup.

Recipe 2:

Moroccan Barley and Lentil Soup

Information about Nutrition:
- 280 calories each serving
- 15g of protein
- 50g of carbohydrates
- 3g of fat
- One and a half hours for cooking
- 6" serving size

Components:
- One cup of washed red lentils

- 1/2 cup of barley pearls
- One chopped onion
- 2 sliced carrots
- Two sliced celery stalks
- Three minced garlic cloves
– Six cups broth made of vegetables
- One teaspoon of cumin powder
- One teaspoon of coriander powder
- Half a teaspoon of ground cinnamon
To taste, add salt and pepper.
- To garnish, fresh cilantro

Guidelines:
1. Lentils, barley, onion, carrots, celery, garlic, vegetable broth, cumin, coriander, and cinnamon should all be combined in a big saucepan. Over high heat, bring the mixture to a boil.
2. Once the lentils and barley are soft, reduce the heat to low, cover the pot, and simmer for one hour.
3. Add salt and pepper to taste when preparing the soup.
4. Spoon soup into bowls; sprinkle with cilantro, if using.
5. Warm Moroccan lentil and barley soup should be served.

Recipe 3:

Barley and Creamy Lentil Soup

Information about Nutrition:
320 calories each serving
14g of protein
- 55g of carbohydrates

- 6g of fat
- One and a half hours for cooking
- 6" serving size

Components:
- One cup of washed brown lentils
- 1/2 cup of barley pearls
- One chopped onion
- 2 sliced carrots
- Two sliced celery stalks
- Three minced garlic cloves
– Six cups broth made of vegetables
- One cup of whole milk
- Two teaspoons of butter
To taste, add salt and pepper.
- Garnish with fresh thyme

Guidelines:
1. Lentils, barley, celery, carrots, onion, garlic, and vegetable broth should all be combined in a big saucepan. Over high heat, bring the mixture to a boil.
2. Once the lentils and barley are soft, reduce the heat to low, cover the pot, and simmer for one hour.
3. Heat the milk and butter in a separate small pot over low heat until the butter melts.
4. Add salt and pepper to taste and stir the milk mixture into the soup.
5. Spoon the rich barley and lentil soup into individual bowls and sprinkle with the fresh thyme.
6. Warm up the soup and serve it.

Recipe 4:

Hot Barley and Lentil Soup

Information about Nutrition:
- 290 calories each serving
13g of protein
- 52g of carbohydrates
- 4g of fat
- One and a half hours for cooking
- 6" serving size

Components:
- One cup of rinsed yellow lentils
- 1/2 cup of barley pearls
- One chopped onion
- 2 sliced carrots
- Two sliced celery stalks
- Three minced garlic cloves
– Six cups broth made of vegetables
- One teaspoon of cayenne pepper, ground
One tsp of paprika
- Half a teaspoon of ground turmeric
To taste, add salt and pepper.
- To garnish, fresh cilantro

Guidelines:
1. Lentils, barley, onion, carrots, celery, garlic, vegetable broth, paprika, cayenne, and turmeric should all be combined in a big saucepan. Over high heat, bring the mixture to a boil.

2. Once the lentils and barley are soft, reduce the heat to low, cover the pot, and simmer for one hour.
3. Add salt and pepper to taste when preparing the soup.
4. Spoon soup into bowls; sprinkle with cilantro, if using.
5. Warm lentil and barley soup should be served spicy.

High-fiber, high-protein beverages

Fruity protein shake

Recipe 1:

Protein Smoothie with Mixed Berries

Information about Nutrition:
- 200 calories each serving
20g of protein
- 25g of carbohydrates
- Fat: 2 g
Cooking Period: Five Minutes
- One serving size

Components:
- One cup of mixed berries, comprising raspberries, blueberries, and strawberries
- A single scoop of vanilla protein powder

- One cup of almond milk without sugar
- One tablespoon of almond butter
- One teaspoon honey, if desired
- Ice cubes, if desired

Guidelines:
1. Blend the almond milk, almond butter, protein powder, mixed berries, and honey (if using) in a blender.
2. Process at high speed until creamy and smooth.
3. If you'd like, add ice cubes and process the smoothie once more to get the consistency you want.
4. Transfer the protein smoothie with mixed berries into a glass and serve right away.

Recipe 2:

Protein Shake with Strawberries and Bananas

Information about Nutrition:
- Each serving has 220 calories.
- 18g of protein
- 30g of carbohydrates
- 3g of fat
Cooking Period: Five Minutes
- One serving size

Components:
- One cup of strawberries, frozen
- One mature banana
- A single scoop of vanilla protein powder

- One cup of almond milk without sugar
Meals: 1 tablespoon of flaxseed
- Ice cubes, if desired

Guidelines:
1. In a blender, combine the frozen strawberries, banana, almond milk, protein powder, and flax seeds.
2. Process at a high speed until all the components are smooth and well blended.
3. If you'd like, add ice cubes and process the smoothie once more to get the consistency you want.
4. Transfer the protein smoothie with strawberries and bananas into a glass and serve right away.

Recipe 3:

Protein Shake with Blueberries and Spinach

Information about Nutrition:
- 180 calories each serving
- 15g of protein
- 25g of carbohydrates
- 4g of fat
Cooking Period: Five Minutes
- One serving size

Components:
- One cup of blueberries, frozen
- One cup of raw spinach
- A single scoop of vanilla protein powder

- One cup of almond milk without sugar
One-third cup chia seeds
- Ice cubes, if desired

Guidelines:
1. In a blender, combine the frozen blueberries, chia seeds, protein powder, spinach leaves, and almond milk.
2. Blend at a high speed until the smoothie is creamy and thoroughly mixed.
3. If you'd like, add ice cubes and combine the smoothie once more to get the thickness you want.
4. Transfer the protein smoothie with spinach and blueberries into a glass and serve right away.

Recipe 4:

Protein Smoothie with Raspberry and Chocolate

Information about Nutrition:
- Each serving has 230 calories.
22g of protein
- 25g of carbohydrates
- 5g of fat
Cooking Period: Five Minutes
- One serving size

Components:
- One cup of raspberries, frozen
1-spoon of chocolate-flavored protein powder
- One cup of almond milk without sugar

- One tablespoon of almond butter
- One tablespoon powdered cocoa
- Ice cubes, if desired

Guidelines:
1. In a blender, combine the cocoa powder, almond butter, almond milk, frozen raspberries, and chocolate protein powder.
2. Blend at a high speed until the smoothie is smooth and all the components are well blended.
3. If you'd like, add ice cubes and process the smoothie once more to get the consistency you want.
4. Transfer the protein smoothie with chocolate and raspberries into a glass and serve right away.

Green power smoothie

Recipe 1:

Traditional Green Power Smoothie

Information about Nutrition:
- 180 calories each serving
- 5g of protein
- 30g of carbohydrates
- 6g of fat
Cooking Period: Five Minutes
- One serving size

Components:
- One cup of spinach leaves
- One mature banana
- Half a cup of cucumber, cut.
- Half a cup of chopped pineapple
- Half a cup of almond milk without sugar
One-third cup chia seeds
- Ice cubes, if desired

Guidelines:
1. Put the spinach leaves, chia seeds, almond milk, banana, cucumber, and pineapple in a blender.
2. Blend at a high speed until the smoothie is smooth and all the components are well blended.
3. If you'd like, add ice cubes and process the smoothie once more to get the consistency you want.
4. Serve the traditional green power smoothie right away after pouring it into a glass.

Recipe 2:

Green Power Smoothie (Tropical)

Information about Nutrition:
- 200 calories each serving
Six grams of protein
- 35g of carbohydrates
- 7g of fat
Cooking Period: Five Minutes
- One serving size

Components:
- One cup of spinach leaves
- Half a cup of diced mango
- Half a cup of chopped pineapple
Half of a ripe avocado
- One cup of coconut water
- One lime's juice
- Ice cubes, if desired

Guidelines:
1. Put the avocado, mango, pineapple, coconut water, lime juice, and spinach leaves in a blender.
2. Blend at a high speed until the smoothie is creamy and all the components are well blended.
3. If you'd like, add ice cubes and combine the smoothie once more to get the thickness you want.
4. Serve the tropical green power smoothie right away after pouring it into a glass.

Recipe 3:

Green Power Smoothie with Berries

Information about Nutrition:
- 160 calories each serving
- 4g of protein
- 30g of carbohydrates
- 5g of fat
Cooking Period: Five Minutes

- One serving size

Components:
- One cup of spinach leaves
- 1/2 cup of mixed berries, including raspberries, blueberries, and strawberries
- One mature banana
- Half a cup of almond milk without sugar
- One tablespoon of almond butter
- Ice cubes, if desired

Guidelines:
1. In a blender, combine the almond milk, almond butter, banana, mixed berries, and spinach leaves.
2. Blend at a high speed until the smoothie is smooth and all the components are well blended.
3. If you'd like, add ice cubes and process the smoothie once more to get the consistency you want.
4. Serve the berry green power smoothie right away after pouring it into a glass.

Recipe 4:

Power Smoothie with Green Protein

Information about Nutrition:
- Each serving has 220 calories.
20g of protein
- 25g of carbohydrates
- 7g of fat

Cooking Period: Five Minutes
- One serving size

Components:
- One cup of spinach leaves
- One mature banana
- A single scoop of vanilla protein powder
- One tablespoon of almond butter
- One cup of almond milk without sugar
- One tablespoon honey, if desired
- Ice cubes, if desired

Guidelines:
1. Put the almond butter, almond milk, protein powder, spinach leaves, banana, and honey (if using) in a blender.
2. Blend at a high speed until the smoothie is creamy and all the components are well blended.
3. If you'd like, add ice cubes and combine the smoothic once more to get the thickness you want.
4. Serve the green protein power smoothie right away after pouring it into a glass.

Berry smoothie with avocado

Recipe 1:

Traditional Berry and Avocado Smoothie

Information about Nutrition:
- Each serving has 220 calories.
- 5g of protein
- 30g of carbohydrates
- 11g of fat
Cooking Period: Five Minutes
- One serving size

Components:
Half of a ripe avocado
- 1/2 cup of mixed berries, including raspberries, blueberries, and strawberries
- One mature banana
- 1 cup unsweetened almond milk
- One tablespoon honey, if desired
- Ice cubes, if desired

Guidelines:
1. Halve the avocado, remove the pit, then scoop out the flesh to put in a blender.
2. In the blender, add the mixed berries, banana, almond milk, and honey (if using).
3. Blend at a high speed until the smoothie is creamy and all the components are well blended.
4. If you'd like, add ice cubes and process the smoothie once more to get the consistency you want.
5. Serve the traditional avocado-berry smoothie right away after pouring it into a glass.

Recipe 2:

Berry-Green Avocado Smoothie

Information about Nutrition:
- 200 calories each serving
Six grams of protein
- 30g of carbohydrates
- 8g of fat
Cooking Period: Five Minutes
- One serving size

Components:
Half of a ripe avocado
- One cup of spinach leaves
- 1/2 cup of mixed berries, including raspberries, blueberries, and strawberries
- One mature banana
- One cup of coconut water
- Ice cubes, if desired

Guidelines:
1. Halve the avocado, remove the pit, then scoop out the flesh to put in a blender.
2. To the blender, add the banana, mixed berries, spinach leaves, and coconut water.
3. Blend at a high speed until the smoothie is smooth and all the components are well blended.
4. If you'd like, add ice cubes and combine the smoothie once more to get the thickness you want.

5. Serve the green avocado berry smoothie right away after pouring it into a glass.

Recipe 3:

Berry-Avocado Tropical Smoothie

Information about Nutrition:
- Each serving has 240 calories.
- 5g of protein
- 35g of carbohydrates
- 10g of fat
Cooking Period: Five Minutes
- One serving size

Components:
Half of a ripe avocado
- 1/2 cup of mixed berries, including raspberries, blueberries, and strawberries
- Half a cup of diced mango
- Half a cup of chopped pineapple
- One cup of orange juice
- Ice cubes, if desired

Guidelines:
1. Halve the avocado, remove the pit, then scoop out the flesh to put in a blender.
2. In the blender, add the orange juice, mango, pineapple, and mixed berries.

3. Blend at a high speed until the smoothie is creamy and all the components are well blended.

4. If you'd like, add ice cubes and process the smoothie once more to get the consistency you want.

5. Serve the tropical avocado berry smoothic right away after pouring it into a glass.

Recipe 4:

Berry Smoothie with Chocolate and Avocado

Information about Nutrition:
- 250 calories per serving.
- 8g of protein
- 35g of carbohydrates
- 12g of fat
Cooking Period: Five Minutes
- One serving size

Components:
Half of a ripe avocado
- 1/2 cup of mixed berries, including raspberries, blueberries, and strawberries
- One mature banana
1-spoon of chocolate-flavored protein powder
- 1 cup unsweetened almond milk
- Ice cubes, if desired

Guidelines:

1. Halve the avocado, remove the pit, then scoop out the flesh to put in a blender.

2. In the blender, add the almond milk, banana, protein powder, and mixed berries.

3. Blend at a high speed until the smoothie is creamy and all the components are well blended.

4. If you'd like, add ice cubes and combine the smoothie once more to get the thickness you want.

5. Serve the chocolate avocado berry smoothie right away after pouring it into a glass.

Iced coffee with protein

Recipe 1:

Iced Coffee with Classic Protein

Information about Nutrition:
- 150 calories each serving
- 15g of protein
- 10g of carbohydrates
- 3g of fat
Cooking Period: Five Minutes
- One serving size

Components:
- One cup of chilled brewed coffee
- A single scoop of vanilla protein powder
- Half a cup of almond milk without sugar

One to two teaspoons of your preferred sweetener (such as sugar, stevia, or honey)
Cubes of ice

Guidelines:
1. The brewed coffee, almond milk, vanilla protein powder, and sweetener should all be combined in a shaker bottle or blender.
2. Once all of the ingredients are well blended and the protein powder has completely dissolved, shake or blend the mixture.
3. Pour the protein coffee mixture over the ice cubes in a glass.
4. Mix thoroughly and taste to adjust the sweetness.
5. Enjoy the traditional protein iced coffee right away after serving.

Recipe 2:

Iced Coffee with Mocha Protein

Information about Nutrition:
- 180 calories each serving
- 15g of protein
- 15g of carbohydrates
- 4g of fat
Cooking Period: Five Minutes
- One serving size

Components:
- One cup of chilled brewed coffee
1-spoon of chocolate-flavored protein powder
- Half a cup of almond milk without sugar
- One tablespoon of powdered unsweetened cocoa

One to two teaspoons of your preferred sweetener (such as sugar, stevia, or honey)
Cubes of ice

Guidelines:
1. The brewed coffee, almond milk, chocolate protein powder, cocoa powder, and sweetener should all be combined in a shaker bottle or blender.
2. Once all of the ingredients are thoroughly mixed and the protein and cocoa powders have completely dissolved, shake or blend the concoction.
3. Pour the mocha protein coffee mixture over the ice cubes in a glass.
4. Mix thoroughly and taste to adjust the sweetness.
5. Enjoy the mocha protein iced coffee right away after serving.

Recipe 3:

Iced Coffee with Vanilla Almond Protein

Information about Nutrition:
- 160 calories each serving
- 15g of protein
- 12g of carbohydrates
- 4g of fat
Cooking Period: Five Minutes
- One serving size

Components:
- One cup of chilled brewed coffee
- A single scoop of vanilla protein powder
- Half a cup of almond milk without sugar

- One-fourth teaspoon almond extract
One to two teaspoons of your preferred sweetener (such as sugar, stevia, or honey)
Cubes of ice

Guidelines:
1. The brewed coffee, almond milk, almond extract, sweetener, and vanilla protein powder should all be combined in a shaker bottle or blender.
2. Once all of the ingredients are well blended and the protein powder has completely dissolved, shake or blend the mixture.
3. Pour the vanilla almond protein coffee concoction over the ice cubes in a glass.
4. Mix thoroughly and taste to adjust the sweetness.
5. Enjoy your vanilla almond protein iced coffee right away after serving.

Recipe 4:

Iced Coffee with Caramel Macchiato Protein

Information about Nutrition:
- 180 calories each serving
- 15g of protein
- 15g of carbohydrates
- 4g of fat
Cooking Period: Five Minutes
- One serving size

Components:
- One cup of chilled brewed coffee
- One scoop of protein powder, caramel

- Half a cup of almond milk without sugar
One to two teaspoons of your preferred sweetener (such as sugar, stevia, or honey)
Cubes of ice
- Caramel sauce with whipped cream as garnish (optional)

Guidelines:
1. The brewed coffee, almond milk, caramel protein powder, and sweetener should all be combined in a shaker bottle or blender.
2. Once all of the ingredients are well blended and the protein powder has completely dissolved, shake or blend the mixture.
3. Pour the protein coffee mixture for the caramel macchiato over the ice cubes in a glass.
4. Mix thoroughly and taste to adjust the sweetness.
5. For extra decadence, you can optionally top with whipped cream and drizzle with caramel sauce.
6. Enjoy the protein iced coffee with caramel macchiato right away.

Dips Hummus and recipes for sauces

Greek yogurt with a dab of dill

Recipe 1:

Dill Dip with Classic Greek Yogurt

Information about Nutrition:
- 60 calories each serving
- 5g of protein
- 3g of carbohydrates
- 3g of fat
- 10 minutes for cooking
Serving Measurement: two tablespoons

Components:
- One cup of Greek yogurt
- Two tablespoons of freshly chopped dill
- One tablespoon of juiced lemon
- One minced garlic clove
To taste, add salt and pepper.

Guidelines:
1. Greek yogurt, minced garlic, lemon juice, chopped dill, salt, and pepper should all be combined in a bowl.
2. Once all the ingredients are well combined, give it a good stir.
3. If necessary, taste and adjust the seasoning by adding extra salt, pepper, or lemon juice to suit your tastes.
4. To enable the flavors to mingle, transfer the dip to a serving bowl and place it in the refrigerator for at least half an hour.
5. Serve this traditional Greek yogurt and dill dip with pita bread, over grilled meats, or with fresh veggies. Have fun!

Recipe 2:

Dill Dip with Spicy Greek Yogurt

Information about Nutrition:
- Each serving has 70 calories.
- 5g of protein
- 4g of carbohydrates
- 4g of fat
- 10 minutes for cooking
Serving Measurement: two tablespoons

Components:
- One cup of Greek yogurt
- Two tablespoons of freshly chopped dill
- One tablespoon of juiced lemon
- One minced garlic clove
- One-half teaspoon of cayenne
To taste, add salt and pepper.

Guidelines:
1. Greek yogurt, chopped dill, lemon juice, minced garlic, cayenne pepper, salt, and pepper should all be combined in a bowl.
2. Until all the ingredients are well incorporated, mix well.
3. If necessary, add additional salt, pepper, or cayenne pepper for greater spiciness after tasting and adjusting the seasoning.
4. To enable the flavors to meld, move the dip to a serving bowl and place it in the refrigerator for at least half an hour.
5. Serve your favorite hot foods alongside the spicy Greek yogurt and dill dip, or use it as a dip for chips and crackers. Savor the kick!

Recipe 3:

Greek yogurt dip with cucumber and dill

Information about Nutrition:
- Each serving has 70 calories.
- 5g of protein
- 6g of carbohydrates
- 3g of fat
- 15 minutes for cooking
Serving Measurement: two tablespoons

Components:
- One cup of Greek yogurt
- Half a cup of grated cucumber, pressed to get rid of extra moisture
- Two tablespoons of freshly chopped dill
- One tablespoon of juiced lemon
- One minced garlic clove
To taste, add salt and pepper.

Guidelines:
1. Greek yogurt, grated cucumber (squeeze out extra moisture), chopped dill, lemon juice, minced garlic, salt, and pepper should all be combined in a bowl.
2. Until all of the ingredients are well combined, mix well.
3. If necessary, taste and adjust the seasoning by adding additional salt, pepper, or lemon juice to suit your taste.
4. To let the flavors combine and the dip thicken, leave it in the fridge for at least an hour.
5. Serve the chilled Greek yogurt dip with cucumber and dill with pita bread or as a side dish for fresh veggies or grilled meats.

Recipe 4:

Greek yogurt dip with avocado and dill

Information about Nutrition:
- 90 calories each serving
- 5g of protein
- 5g of carbohydrates
- 6g of fat
- 10 minutes for cooking
Serving Measurement: two tablespoons

Components:
- One mature avocado, pitted and peeled
- One cup of Greek yogurt
- Two tablespoons of freshly chopped dill
- One tablespoon of juiced lemon
- One minced garlic clove
To taste, add salt and pepper.

Guidelines:
1. Use a fork to mash the ripe avocado in a bowl until it becomes smooth.
2. To the mashed avocado, add the Greek yogurt, minced garlic, lemon juice, chopped dill, salt, and pepper.
3. Make sure all the ingredients are fully blended by giving it a good stir.
4. If necessary, adjust the seasoning by tasting and adding additional salt, pepper, or lemon juice.
5. To give the flavors time to meld, move the Greek yogurt dip with avocado and dill to a serving bowl and place it in the refrigerator for at least half an hour.

6. Serve the rich and creamy Greek yogurt dip with avocado and dill on sandwiches or as a dip for veggie sticks or tortilla chips. Savor the delicious creaminess!

Hot Red Pepper Hummus

Recipe 1:

Traditional Hot Red Pepper Hummus

Information about Nutrition:
- Each serving has 70 calories.
- 3g of protein
- 8g of carbohydrates
- 3g of fat
- 10 minutes for cooking
Serving Measurement: two tablespoons

Components:
One can (15 ounces) of rinsed and drained chickpeas
- 1/4 cup of drained roasted red peppers
– Two teaspoons of tahini
- One minced garlic clove
- Half a cup of lemon juice
A tsp of olive oil
- Half a teaspoon of cumin
One-fourth teaspoon cayenne pepper, or to taste
- To taste salt

Guidelines:

1. The chickpeas, tahini, minced garlic, lemon juice, olive oil, cumin, cayenne pepper, and salt should all be combined in a food processor.

2. Blend the blend till it becomes creamy and smooth. To get the right consistency, add a little water, one tablespoon at a time, if necessary.

3. Add extra lemon juice, cayenne pepper, or salt to taste and adjust the seasoning accordingly.

4. Move the hot red pepper hummus into a dish for serving.

5. Serve the hummus as a spread for sandwiches or as an accompaniment to pita bread or vegetable sticks. Have fun!

Recipe 2:

Red pepper hummus with smoky chipotles

Information about Nutrition:
- 80 calories a serving
- 3g of protein
- 9g of carbohydrates
- 4g of fat
- 10 minutes for cooking
Serving Measurement: two tablespoons

Components:
One can (15 ounces) of rinsed and drained chickpeas
- 1/4 cup of drained roasted red peppers
– Two teaspoons of tahini
- One minced garlic clove
- Half a cup of lemon juice
A tsp of olive oil

- One teaspoon finely chopped chipotle pepper in adobo sauce
- To taste salt

Guidelines:
1. Chickpeas, roasted red peppers, tahini, minced garlic, lemon juice, olive oil, chipotle pepper, and salt should all be combined in a food processor.
2. Blend the blend till it becomes creamy and smooth. If needed, thin out the consistency with a small amount of water.
3. Add extra salt, chipotle pepper, or lemon juice to taste and adjust the seasoning accordingly.
4. Spoon the chipotle red pepper hummus over a serving bowl to release the smoke.
5. Serve the hummus as a tasty veggie dip or with pita bread or tortilla chips. Savor the kick of smoke!

Recipe 3:

Roasted Red Pepper and Garlic Hummus

Information about Nutrition:
- 90 calories each serving
- 3g of protein
- 9g of carbohydrates
- 5g of fat
- 20 minutes for cooking
Serving Measurement: two tablespoons

Components:
One can (15 ounces) of rinsed and drained chickpeas
- 1/4 cup of drained roasted red peppers

– Two teaspoons of tahini
- One head of garlic
- Half a cup of lemon juice
A tsp of olive oil
- To taste salt

Guidelines:
1. Set oven temperature to 400°F, or 200°C.
2. Cut the top of the garlic head off so that the cloves are visible.
3. After lightly oiling the garlic head, put it on a baking pan and cover it with aluminum foil.
4. Bake the garlic for about 20 minutes, or until the cloves are tender and golden, in a preheated oven.
5. After taking the roasted garlic out of the oven, allow it to cool a little.
6. Add the tahini, lemon juice, olive oil, roasted red peppers, chickpeas, and a dash of salt to a food processor.
7. Add the roasted garlic cloves to the food processor after squeezing them free of their shells.
8. Blend the ingredients until it's creamy and smooth, adding a little water if necessary to alter the consistency.
9. If needed, add extra salt or lemon juice after tasting and adjusting the seasoning.
Ten. Move the red pepper hummus with roasted garlic to a serving bowl.
11. Serve the hummus as a delicious spread on sandwiches or alongside pita bread and breadsticks. Savor the flavor of the rich garlic!

Recipe 4:

Red pepper, lime, and jalapeño hummus

Information about Nutrition:
- 80 calories a serving
- 3g of protein
- 10g of carbohydrates
- 4g of fat
- 10 minutes for cooking
Serving Measurement: two tablespoons

Components:
One can (15 ounces) of rinsed and drained chickpeas
- 1/4 cup of drained roasted red peppers
– Two teaspoons of tahini
- One minced garlic clove
- Two teaspoons of juiced lime
A tsp of olive oil
- One jalapeño pepper, chopped and seeded
- To taste salt

Guidelines:
1. The chickpeas, tahini, minced garlic, lime juice, olive oil, minced jalapeño pepper, and salt should all be combined in a food processor.
2. Blend the blend till it becomes creamy and smooth. If needed, dilute the consistency with a small amount of water.
3. To suit your taste, add additional salt or lime juice after tasting and adjusting the seasoning.
4. Move the red pepper hummus with jalapeño and lime to a serving bowl.
5. Serve the hummus as a spicy spread on wraps, alongside vegetable sticks or tortilla chips. Savor the hint of lime with a fiery bite!

Garlic roasted in Tzatziki

Recipe 1:

Traditional Tzatziki with Roasted Garlic

Information about Nutrition:
- 60 calories each serving
- 4g of protein
- 5g of carbohydrates
- 3g of fat
- 1 hour and fifteen minutes of cooking time (this includes roasting the garlic)

Serving Measurement: two tablespoons

Components:
- One cup of Greek yogurt
- Half a cucumber, grated, then squeezed to get rid of extra water
- One head of garlic
- One tablespoon of juiced lemon

A tsp of extra virgin olive oil
- One tablespoon of freshly chopped dill

To taste, add salt and pepper.

Guidelines:
1. Set oven temperature to 400°F, or 200°C.
2. Cut the top of the garlic head off so that the cloves are visible.
3. After lightly oiling the garlic head, put it on a baking pan and cover it with aluminum foil.

4. Roast the garlic for 45 to 1 hour, or until the cloves are tender and golden, in an oven that has been warmed.

5. After taking the roasted garlic out of the oven, allow it to cool a little.

6. Greek yogurt, grated cucumber, extra virgin olive oil, minced dill, lemon juice, salt, and pepper should all be combined in a bowl.

7. Add the roasted garlic cloves to the bowl after squeezing them out of their shells.

8. Until all the ingredients are well incorporated, mix well.

9. If needed, add extra lemon juice, salt, or pepper after tasting and adjusting the seasoning.

Ten. To let the flavors settle, place the tzatziki in the refrigerator for at least an hour.

11. Serve the traditional tzatziki made with roasted garlic with pita bread, salad dressing, or as a condiment for grilled meats. Savor the tasty and creamy dip!

Recipe 2:

Roasted Garlic Tzatziki with Dill and Lemon

Information about Nutrition:
- Each serving has 70 calories.
- 4g of protein
- 6g of carbohydrates
- 4g of fat
- 1 hour and fifteen minutes of cooking time (this includes roasting the garlic)
Serving Measurement: two tablespoons

Components:
- One cup of Greek yogurt

- Half a cucumber, grated, then squeezed to get rid of extra water
- One head of garlic
- One tablespoon of juiced lemon
A tsp of extra virgin olive oil
- One tablespoon of freshly chopped dill
- One lemon's zest
To taste, add salt and pepper.

Guidelines:
1. Set oven temperature to 400°F, or 200°C.
2. Cut the top of the garlic head off so that the cloves are visible.
3. After lightly oiling the garlic head, put it on a baking pan and cover it with aluminum foil.
4. Roast the garlic for 45 to 1 hour, or until the cloves are tender and golden, in an oven that has been warmed.
5. After taking the roasted garlic out of the oven, allow it to cool a little.
6. Greek yogurt, grated cucumber, extra virgin olive oil, minced dill, lemon zest, salt, and pepper should all be combined in a bowl.
7. Add the roasted garlic cloves to the bowl after squeezing them out of their shells.
8. Until all the ingredients are well incorporated, mix well.
9. If needed, add extra lemon juice, salt, or pepper after tasting and adjusting the seasoning.
Ten. To allow the flavors to blend, place the dill and lemon-roasted garlic tzatziki in the refrigerator for at least an hour.
11. Serve the zesty tzatziki as a side dish for grilled meats, pita bread, or veggie sticks. Savor the spicy twist!

Recipe 3:

Roasted Garlic Tzatziki with Mint and Cucumber

Information about Nutrition:
- Each serving has 70 calories.
- 4g of protein
- 6g of carbohydrates
- 4g of fat
- 1 hour and fifteen minutes of cooking time (this includes roasting the garlic)
Serving Measurement: two tablespoons

Components:
- One cup of Greek yogurt
- Half a cucumber, grated, then squeezed to get rid of extra water
- One head of garlic
- One tablespoon of juiced lemon
A tsp of extra virgin olive oil
- One tablespoon finely chopped fresh mint
To taste, add salt and pepper.

Guidelines:
1. Set oven temperature to 400°F, or 200°C.
2. Cut the top of the garlic head off so that the cloves are visible.
3. After lightly oiling the garlic head, put it on a baking pan and cover it with aluminum foil.
4. Roast the garlic for 45 to 1 hour, or until the cloves are tender and golden, in an oven that has been warmed.
5. After taking the roasted garlic out of the oven, allow it to cool a little.
6. Greek yogurt, grated cucumber, extra virgin olive oil, chopped mint, lemon juice, salt, and pepper should all be combined in a bowl.

7. Add the roasted garlic cloves to the bowl after squeezing them out of their shells.

8. Until all the ingredients are well incorporated, mix well.

9. If needed, add extra lemon juice, salt, or pepper after tasting and adjusting the seasoning.

10. To allow the flavors to blend, place the cucumber-roasted garlic tzatziki and mint in the refrigerator for at least an hour.

11. Serve the chilled tzatziki as a sauce to cook grilled meats, as a dip for vegetable crudités, or with pita bread. Savor the delicious fusion of garlic and mint!

Recipe 4:

Roasted Garlic Tzatziki with Spices

Information about Nutrition:
- Each serving has 70 calories.
- 4g of protein
- 6g of carbohydrates
- 4g of fat
- 1 hour and fifteen minutes of cooking time (this includes roasting the garlic)
Serving Measurement: two tablespoons

Components:
- One cup of Greek yogurt
- Half a cucumber, grated, then squeezed to get rid of extra water
- One head of garlic
- One tablespoon of juiced lemon
A tsp of extra virgin olive oil

- One tablespoon of freshly chopped parsley
- 1/2 teaspoon (or more, depending on taste) red pepper flakes
To taste, add salt and pepper.

Guidelines:
1. Set oven temperature to 400°F, or 200°C.
2. Cut the top of the garlic head off so that the cloves are visible.
3. After lightly oiling the garlic head, put it on a baking pan and cover it with aluminum foil.
4. Roast the garlic for 45 to 1 hour, or until the cloves are tender and golden, in an oven that has been warmed.
5. After taking the roasted garlic out of the oven, allow it to cool a little.
6. Greek yogurt, grated cucumber, extra virgin olive oil, chopped parsley, red pepper flakes, salt, and pepper should all be combined in a bowl.
7. Add the roasted garlic cloves to the bowl after squeezing them out of their shells.
8. Until all the ingredients are well incorporated, mix well.
9. To suit your taste, add additional lemon juice, red pepper flakes, salt, or pepper to the seasoning.
Ten. To let the flavors combine, place the spicy roasted garlic tzatziki in the refrigerator for a minimum of one hour.
11. Serve the spicy tzatziki as a dip for grilled meats, as a condiment for sandwiches, or with pita bread. Savor the blast of spice in this tasty dip!

Corn salsa with avocados

Recipe 1:

Traditional Corn and Avocado Salsa

Information about Nutrition:
- 80 calories a serving
- 2g of protein
- 10g of carbohydrates
- 5g of fat
- 15 minutes for cooking
Portion Size: half a cup

Components:
- One cup of frozen or fresh corn kernels
- One diced avocado
- Half a red onion, diced finely
- One jalapeño jalapeno, seeded and cut finely
- One sliced tomato
- One lime's juice
- 2 teaspoons finely chopped fresh cilantro
To taste, add salt and pepper.

Guidelines:
1. Cook the corn kernels in boiling water for three to four minutes if you're using fresh corn. Thaw frozen corn as directed on the packaging if using it.
2. The cooked corn, diced avocado, red onion, jalapeño pepper, and diced tomato should all be combined in a bowl.
3. Add the chopped cilantro to the mixture after adding the juice from one lime.
4. To taste, add salt and pepper for seasoning.
5. Mix all the ingredients together gently until thoroughly mixed.
6. To allow the flavors to mingle, let the salsa sit at room temperature for approximately ten minutes before serving.

7. Serve this traditional salsa of avocado and corn as a topping for salads, tacos, and grilled meats. It can also be served as a dip with tortilla chips. Savor the flavors that are bright and fresh!

Recipe 2:

Avocado and Black Bean Corn Salsa

Information about Nutrition:
- 120 calories per serving.
- 4g of protein
- 18g of carbohydrates
- 5g of fat
- 15 minutes for cooking
Portion Size: half a cup

Components:
- One cup of frozen or fresh corn kernels
- One diced avocado
- Half a red onion, diced finely
- One jalapeño jalapeno, seeded and cut finely
- One sliced tomato
- One cup of washed and drained black beans
- One lime's juice
- 2 teaspoons finely chopped fresh cilantro
To taste, add salt and pepper.

Guidelines:
1. Cook the corn kernels in boiling water for three to four minutes if you're using fresh corn. Thaw frozen corn as directed on the packaging if using it.

2. Cooked corn, diced avocado, red onion, jalapeño pepper, diced tomato, and black beans should all be combined in a bowl.
3. Add the chopped cilantro to the mixture after adding the juice from one lime.
4. To taste, add salt and pepper for seasoning.
5. Mix all the ingredients together gently until thoroughly mixed.
6. To allow the flavors to mingle, let the salsa sit at room temperature for approximately ten minutes before serving.
7. Serve the avocado and black bean corn salsa as a tasty topping for tacos, quesadillas, or grilled chicken, or as a dip with tortilla chips. Savor the mouthwatering fusion of tastes and textures!

Recipe 3:

Corn salsa with mango and avocado

Information about Nutrition:
- 100 calories each serving
- 2g of protein
- 18g of carbohydrates
- 5g of fat
- 15 minutes for cooking
Portion Size: half a cup

Components:
- One cup of frozen or fresh corn kernels
- One diced avocado
- One chopped mango
- Half a red onion, diced finely
- One jalapeño jalapeno, seeded and cut finely

- One lime's juice
- 2 teaspoons finely chopped fresh cilantro
To taste, add salt and pepper.

Guidelines:
1. Cook the corn kernels in boiling water for three to four minutes if you're using fresh corn. Thaw frozen corn as directed on the packaging if using it.
2. The cooked corn, diced mango, diced avocado, finely sliced red onion, and jalapeño pepper should all be combined in a bowl.
3. Add the chopped cilantro to the mixture after adding the juice from one lime.
4. To taste, add salt and pepper for seasoning.
5. Mix all the ingredients together gently until thoroughly mixed.
6. To allow the flavors to mingle, let the salsa sit at room temperature for approximately ten minutes before serving.
7. Serve the mango and avocado corn salsa as a tropical garnish for salads, fish tacos, or grilled shrimp. It can also be served as a cool dip with tortilla chips. Savor the flavors that are tart and sweet!

Recipe 4:

Corn salsa with tomatoes and avocado

Information about Nutrition:
- 90 calories each serving
- 2g of protein
- 12g of carbohydrates
- 5g of fat
- 15 minutes for cooking
Portion Size: half a cup

Components:
- One cup of frozen or fresh corn kernels
- One diced avocado
- One sliced tomato
- Half a red onion, diced finely
- One jalapeño jalapeno, seeded and cut finely
- One lime's juice
- 2 teaspoons finely chopped fresh cilantro
To taste, add salt and pepper.

Guidelines:
1. Cook the corn kernels in boiling water for three to four minutes if you're using fresh corn. Thaw frozen corn as directed on the packaging if using it.
2. The cooked corn, diced avocado, diced tomato, finely sliced red onion, and jalapeño pepper should all be combined in a bowl.
3. Add the chopped cilantro to the mixture after adding the juice from one lime.
4. To taste, add salt and pepper for seasoning.
5. Mix all the ingredients together gently until thoroughly mixed.
6. To allow the flavors to mingle, let the salsa sit at room temperature for approximately ten minutes before serving.
7. Use the tomato and avocado corn salsa as a topping for tacos, quesadillas, grilled chicken, or even scrambled eggs. It may also be served as a flexible dip with tortilla chips. Savor the flavors that are bright and zesty!

Meal planning: Set aside some time at the start of each week to organize your meals. Think about including a range of high-protein and high-fiber foods, such as fish, poultry, beans, lentils, whole grains, fruits, and vegetables, as well as lean meats. This will guarantee that your meal plan is wholesome and well-balanced.

Batch cooking and portion control: Make bigger batches of recipes that are high in fiber and protein and then portion them out into serving sizes. You'll save time and find it simpler to get a nutritious lunch when you're pressed for time. For meal prep or portion management, use containers to make sure you're eating the proper amount of food.

Select whole foods: Refrain from using processed foods in favor of entire foods. In general, whole foods are lower in harmful fats and additives and higher in protein and fiber. Include lean protein sources like chicken breast, tofu, and Greek yogurt, whole grains like quinoa, brown rice, and oats, and an abundance of fruits and vegetables.

Include plant-based protein sources in your diet: Take into account including tofu, beans, lentils, and chickpeas in your meals. These choices include important vitamins and minerals in addition to being high in protein and fiber. Try out various recipes to give your meals more taste and diversity.

Although meals high in protein and fiber are good for you, it's still crucial to watch how much you eat. When eaten in excess, even healthful meals can add to weight gain. To be sure you're following suggested serving amounts, use a food scale or measuring cups.

Use herbs and spices: Try incorporating different herbs and spices into your food instead of depending too much on unhealthy sauces or excessive salt. While spices like cumin, paprika, and turmeric can add depth and complexity, fresh herbs like basil, cilantro, and parsley can improve the flavor of your food.

Remain hydrated: Water consumption is essential for healthy digestion and general well-being. Water is necessary for high-fiber foods to pass through the digestive system efficiently. In order to aid with digestion and maintain proper hydration, try to consume at least 8 cups (64 ounces) of water each day.

Follow good food storage practices: To preserve the freshness and quality of your meal-prepared goods, make sure they are stored correctly. Purchase airtight receptacles and freeze or chill your meals as needed. Put a date on the containers so you can monitor their freshness and make sure you eat them within the suggested time limit.

After eating meals heavy in protein and fiber, pay attention to how your body feels. This is known as listening to your body. Since each person has unique dietary requirements and tolerances, it's critical to pay attention to your body's cues. As necessary, modify your meal plan to fit your unique requirements and tastes.

Consult a qualified dietitian or other healthcare provider if necessary: It's always a good idea to speak with someone about unique dietary needs, medical conditions, or concerns. They can offer you individualized advice and make sure your high-protein, high-fiber meal preparation is in line with your objectives and general wellbeing.

CONCLUSION

Including meal prep that is high in protein and high in fiber in your routine is a wise and long-lasting approach to help you achieve your wellness and health objectives. You can make sure that you're providing your body with a balanced and nutritious diet by organizing your meals, cooking in large quantities, and watching how much food you eat. Your meal prep should be built around whole foods, such as whole grains, lean protein sources, and an abundance of fruits and vegetables.

To increase diversity and lessen dependency on processed substitutes, it's critical to pay attention to portion sizes and select plant-based protein sources. Adding different herbs and spices to your food will help you to improve its flavor without sacrificing its nutritional value. To preserve freshness, digestion, and general wellbeing, it's critical to store food properly, stay hydrated, and pay attention to your body's signals.

Recall that achievement and sustainability result from striking a balance that suits you. A licensed dietician or other healthcare expert can offer individualized counsel if you have any unique dietary needs or concerns. You can experience better nutrition, more energy, and general health by adopting the high-protein, high-fiber meal prep strategy.

So begin meal planning, restock on healthful products, and set out on a path to a more energetic and health-conscious lifestyle by preparing meals that are high in protein and fiber. You'll be on the road to long-term success and wellbeing, and your body will thank you for the nutrients and attention it receives.

31 Days Meal Plan

Day	Breakfast	Lunch	Dinner	Snack
1	Berry Protein Smoothie	Grilled Chicken Breasts	Beef Stir-Fry with Rice	Greek Yogurt and Dill Dip with Veggies
2	Green Power Smoothie	Lentil and Barley Soup	Chicken Marsala with Quinoa	Avocado and Corn Salsa
3	Protein Iced Coffee	Beef and Vegetable Stew	Avocado Berry Smoothie	Roasted Garlic Tzatziki with Pita
4	Avocado Berry Smoothie	Chicken and Shrimp Paella	Lentil and Vegetable Curry	Spicy Red Pepper Hummus with Crackers
5	Berry Protein Smoothie	Grilled Chicken Breasts	Beef Stir-Fry with Rice	Greek Yogurt and Dill Dip with Veggies

6	Green Power Smoothie	Lentil and Barley Soup	Chicken Marsala with Quinoa	Avocado and Corn Salsa
7	Protein Iced Coffee	Beef and Vegetable Stew	Avocado Berry Smoothie	Roasted Garlic Tzatziki with Pita
8	Avocado Berry Smoothie	Chicken and Shrimp Paella	Lentil and Vegetable Curry	Spicy Red Pepper Hummus with Crackers
9	Berry Protein Smoothie	Grilled Chicken Breasts	Beef Stir-Fry with Rice	Greek Yogurt and Dill Dip with Veggies
10	Green Power Smoothie	Lentil and Barley Soup	Chicken Marsala with Quinoa	Avocado and Corn Salsa
11	Protein Iced Coffee	Beef and Vegetable Stew	Avocado Berry Smoothie	Roasted Garlic Tzatziki with Pita
12	Avocado Berry Smoothie	Chicken and Shrimp Paella	Lentil and Vegetable Curry	Spicy Red Pepper Hummus with Crackers
13	Berry Protein Smoothie	Grilled Chicken Breasts	Beef Stir-Fry with Rice	Greek Yogurt and Dill Dip with Veggies
14	Green Power Smoothie	Lentil and Barley Soup	Chicken Marsala with Quinoa	Avocado and Corn Salsa

15	Protein Iced Coffee	Beef and Vegetable Stew	Avocado Berry Smoothie	Roasted Garlic Tzatziki with Pita
16	Avocado Berry Smoothie	Chicken and Shrimp Paella	Lentil and Vegetable Curry	Spicy Red Pepper Hummus with Crackers
17	Berry Protein Smoothie	Grilled Chicken Breasts	Beef Stir-Fry with Rice	Greek Yogurt and Dill Dip with Veggies
18	Green Power Smoothie	Lentil and Barley Soup	Chicken Marsala with Quinoa	Avocado and Corn Salsa
19	Protein Iced Coffee	Beef and Vegetable Stew	Avocado Berry Smoothie	Roasted Garlic Tzatziki with Pita
20	Avocado Berry Smoothie	Chicken and Shrimp Paella	Lentil and Vegetable Curry	Spicy Red Pepper Hummus with Crackers
21	Berry Protein Smoothie	Grilled Chicken Breasts	Beef Stir-Fry with Rice	Greek Yogurt and Dill Dip with Veggies
22	Green Power Smoothie	Lentil and Barley Soup	Chicken Marsala with Quinoa	Avocado and Corn Salsa
23	Protein Iced Coffee	Beef and Vegetable Stew	Avocado Berry Smoothie	Roasted Garlic Tzatziki with Pita

24	Avocado Berry Smoothie	Chicken and Shrimp Paella	Lentil and Vegetable Curry	Spicy Red Pepper Hummus with Crackers
25	Berry Protein Smoothie	Grilled Chicken Breasts	Beef Stir-Fry with Rice	Greek Yogurt and Dill Dip with Veggies
26	Green Power Smoothie	Lentil and Barley Soup	Chicken Marsala with Quinoa	Avocado and Corn Salsa
27	Protein Iced Coffee	Beef and Vegetable Stew	Avocado Berry Smoothie	Roasted Garlic Tzatziki with Pita
28	Avocado Berry Smoothie	Chicken and Shrimp Paella	Lentil and Vegetable Curry	Spicy Red Pepper Hummus with Crackers
29	Berry Protein Smoothie	Grilled Chicken Breasts	Beef Stir-Fry with Rice	Greek Yogurt and Dill Dip with Veggies
30	Green Power Smoothie	Lentil and Barley Soup	Chicken Marsala with Quinoa	Avocado and Corn Salsa
31	Protein Iced Coffee	Beef and Vegetable Stew	Avocado Berry Smoothie	Roasted Garlic Tzatziki with Pita